TENDER W[

A Compassionate guide to Alzheimer's and Dementia care

By Dr. Elvis Hartmann

Copyright @ 2024 Dr. Elvis Hartmann

Legal Notice

All rights reserved. No part of this book may be reproduced, stored in a retrieval system, or transmitted in any form or by any means, electronic, mechanical, photocopying, recording, or otherwise, without the prior written permission of the copyright owner, except for the use of brief quotations in a book review.

The information provided in this book is for general informational purposes only. While the author has made every effort to ensure the accuracy of the information contained within, the content is not intended as medical, legal, or professional advice. Readers should consult a qualified professional for specific advice concerning their individual circumstances.

The author and publisher disclaim any liability for any direct or indirect damages or losses arising from the use or reliance on any information or strategies presented in this book.

Disclaimer Note

The information in "*Tender Watch: A Compassionate Guide to Alzheimer's and Dementia Care* " is meant to be helpful and informative, but it's not a substitute for professional advice. The insights and suggestions in this book are based on general knowledge and personal stories, and while we strive for accuracy, we can't guarantee that they will apply to every individual situation.

Always consult with healthcare providers, educators, or other professionals when dealing with specific concerns or challenges. The personal success stories shared here reflect individual experiences and may not represent everyone's journey.

We hope you find this book valuable, but please use it as a guide rather than a definitive source. The authors and publisher are not responsible for any outcomes resulting from the use of this book. Thank you for understanding!

Table of Contents

Preface 5

Chapter 1 8

   Introduction: Understanding Alzheimer's and Dementia 8

Chapter 2 15

   Understanding Alzheimer's and Dementia 15

      What is Dementia? 15

      What is Alzheimer's Disease? 16

      Common Risk Factors for Alzheimer's and Dementia 17

Chapter 3 20

   Diagnosis and Stages 20

   The Diagnosis Process 21

   Navigating Medical Appointments 24

   Tips for Caregivers 26

Chapter 4 28

   Treatment and Care Options for Alzheimer's and Dementia 28

   Medications for Alzheimer's and Dementia 28

   Establish a Routine 32

   Creating a Supportive Home Environment 34

Chapter 5 37

Understanding Behavioral Changes in Alzheimer's and Dementia 37

Common Behavioral Challenges and Effective Coping Strategies 38

Supporting the Person and Their Family Emotionally 40

Creating a Supportive Environment 42

Engaging in Activities 42

The Power of Empathy and Patience 43

Chapter 6 44

The Role of Diet in Managing Alzheimer's and Dementia 44

Understanding the Connection Between Diet and Brain Health 44

    Important Nutritional Components for Brain Function: 44

Ideas for Meal Planning 47

Creating a Brain-Healthy Meal Plan 50

Chapter 7 53

Support for Families and Caregivers 53

Coping Strategies for Caregivers 54

Resources for Caregivers 56

Personal Stories of Community and Support 58

Chapter 8 60

A Comprehensive Collection of Expert Insights and
Real-Life Stories on Alzheimer's and Dementia 60

Lessons Learned from Experts 60

The Importance of Self-Care 67

Chapter 9 69

Planning for the Future 69

Understanding the Importance of Planning 69

Legal Considerations 70

Financial Considerations 72

Navigating Complex Topics 75

Chapter 10 78

Conclusion to the Guide on Alzheimer's and
Dementia 78

Preface

Caring for someone with Alzheimer's or dementia is a journey unlike any other. It often brings unexpected challenges that can leave you feeling overwhelmed, frustrated, or lost. Yet, amid the trials, this path also offers profound moments of connection and insight that touch the heart in deep and lasting ways. *Tender Watch: A Compassionate Guide to Alzheimer's and Dementia Care* is here to support you through the emotional ups and downs of caregiving, providing not just information but also comfort and understanding.

The inspiration for this book comes from countless conversations with caregivers who have bravely shared their experiences. I realized that, more than just a guide, we needed a resource that speaks to the heart of what it means to care for someone facing these conditions. The title, *Tender Watch*, reflects this delicate balance—remaining vigilant while also embracing the tenderness that comes from cherishing every moment, even when the challenges feel insurmountable.

In these pages, you'll find a wealth of insights from experts who understand the complexities of dementia care, as well as stories from individuals who have walked this path. Their experiences highlight not only the hurdles but also the unexpected joys that can arise during this journey. You'll learn practical strategies for daily challenges, such as managing behavioral changes, communicating effectively, and creating a nurturing environment that supports your loved one's well-being.

As you read, I encourage you to take a moment to reflect on your own experiences. You may find yourself nodding in agreement with the struggles shared or feeling a sense of relief in knowing that others have faced similar situations. This book is designed to be a companion—a reassuring presence reminding you that you are not alone in this endeavor. It's natural to feel a mix of emotions, from love and compassion to sadness and frustration. Embracing those feelings is part of the journey.

Furthermore, *Tender Watch* emphasizes the importance of self-care for caregivers. You cannot pour from an empty cup, and taking time for yourself is crucial in maintaining the strength and energy needed to provide care. Within these chapters, you'll discover tips on how to prioritize your own well-being while still being there for your loved one.

This guide also aims to foster a sense of community, connecting you with resources, support groups, and networks of others who understand what you're going through. Caregiving can feel isolating, but together, we can create a supportive network that lifts each other up. You are part of a larger story—one that includes many who have faced and continue to face the challenges of Alzheimer's and dementia.

With your loved one, as you set out on this journey , I hope *Tender Watch* serves as a source of strength, encouragement, and empowerment. Your role as a caregiver is invaluable, and the love you bring to this journey is immeasurable. Let this book be a reminder of the compassion, resilience, and love that guide you every step of the way. Embrace the moments of connection, and know that you are making a profound difference in the life of someone you cherish. Together, we can navigate this path with grace, understanding, and hope.

Chapter 1

Introduction: Understanding Alzheimer's and Dementia

When we think about aging, we often imagine the wisdom that comes with years, the stories shared over family dinners, and the memories passed down through generations. However, for some families, the journey of aging takes a challenging turn when Alzheimer's disease or other forms of dementia come into play. These conditions can profoundly affect not just the individuals diagnosed but also their loved ones. Understanding Alzheimer's and dementia is essential for everyone, especially caregivers. This knowledge fosters empathy and helps families navigate the emotional and practical challenges these conditions present.

Dementia itself is an umbrella term used to describe a range of cognitive impairments that interfere with daily life. These impairments can include:

- Memory loss
- Difficulties with communication

- Challenges in reasoning or judgment

While many people associate dementia with old age, it is important to note that it is not a normal part of aging. Conditions like Alzheimer's can develop in people as young as their 30s or 40s, although the risk increases with age.

To illustrate the impact of Alzheimer's and dementia, let's consider the story of the Thompson family. When Jane Thompson first noticed that her husband, Michael, was frequently misplacing items and forgetting recent conversations, she brushed it off as typical aging. After all, Michael was in his late sixties, and everyone experiences "senior moments," right? But as time passed, Jane noticed more concerning signs:

- Michael began to struggle with familiar tasks, such as balancing the checkbook and following recipes.

- The gentle man she had married was becoming more frustrated and withdrawn.

After a heartbreaking trip to the doctor, Jane and Michael received the diagnosis that would change their lives: Alzheimer's disease. The news was devastating. Jane felt a wave of grief wash over her as she realized that the man she loved would slowly fade away. The emotional toll of this diagnosis cannot be overstated. Jane not only grieved for Michael's future but also felt an overwhelming sense of fear about what lay ahead for her as his caregiver.

As she navigated the complexities of caregiving, Jane learned that awareness and understanding were her greatest allies. She began to research Alzheimer's, discovering how the disease progresses and what she could do to support Michael. This awareness helped Jane feel more empowered; she could anticipate challenges and better understand the changes she was witnessing. It also allowed her to develop a sense of empathy towards Michael's struggles. She recognized that he wasn't just being forgetful or stubborn; he was battling a disease that was robbing him of his memories and identity.

In her journey, Jane also found solace in connecting with other caregivers. She joined a local support group, where she met others facing similar challenges. Sharing stories with people who understood her experience provided Jane with a sense of community and validation. She learned that many caregivers experience feelings of guilt, isolation, and burnout. Through these conversations, she discovered practical strategies for self-care and ways to cope with the emotional strain of caregiving.

Empathy is crucial in this journey. Understanding that Alzheimer's is not just about memory loss but involves emotional and psychological changes as well helps caregivers provide better support. For example, when Michael became frustrated because he couldn't find the words to express himself, Jane learned to approach him with patience rather than frustration. She reminded herself that he was scared and confused, not intentionally uncooperative. This shift in perspective helped Jane maintain a positive relationship with Michael, even as the disease progressed.

Another important aspect of caregiving is recognizing the importance of maintaining the dignity of the person with Alzheimer's or dementia It can be difficult to find this equilibrium. For instance, when Michael began to struggle with personal hygiene, Jane faced a difficult decision about how to intervene without making him feel ashamed or embarrassed. She learned to approach these situations delicately, always allowing Michael to maintain as much independence as possible:

- Laying out his clothes in the morning, giving him the choice to dress himself rather than simply taking over the task.

- Encouraging him to brush his teeth and wash his face while providing gentle reminders.

These small gestures helped preserve his dignity and fostered a sense of agency.

As Jane and Michael's journey continued, they faced numerous challenges together, but they also experienced moments of joy. Some days, Michael would surprise Jane by recalling a song from their wedding day or a favorite family vacation. These moments, though fleeting, became cherished memories that reminded Jane of the man she fell in love with. They also served as a reminder to celebrate the small victories, no matter how minor they may seem.

The impact of Alzheimer's and dementia extends beyond the individual diagnosed; it reshapes family dynamics and relationships. Children, siblings, and friends may also struggle with the emotional toll of seeing a loved one change. It's not uncommon for families to feel frustrated, helpless, or angry. The reality is that everyone processes this grief differently, and it's essential for families to communicate openly and support one another through this difficult time.

Consider the story of the Garcia family. When their mother, Rosa, began to show signs of dementia, her adult children initially reacted with denial. They found it hard to believe that their vibrant, strong-willed mother could be losing her memory. However, as they started to notice her confusion and forgetfulness, they were forced to confront the reality of her condition. This confrontation led to heated discussions about her care and future, which, at times, felt overwhelming.

To foster understanding and support, the Garcia siblings decided to hold regular family meetings. These meetings provided a safe space for each member to express their feelings and concerns. They shared their worries about Rosa's safety, the challenges of caregiving, and their hopes for her remaining years. This open dialogue not only strengthened their bond as siblings but also helped them better understand the complexities of dementia and how they could collectively support their mother.

Through these discussions, the Garcias learned about the importance of patience and flexibility. Rosa had her good days and her bad days, and the family found that adjusting their expectations was crucial for maintaining harmony. They discovered the value of small, meaningful moments, such as sharing a cup of tea or reminiscing about family traditions, which brought joy and connection despite the challenges they faced.

As we navigate the emotional journey of Alzheimer's and dementia, it's crucial to recognize the significance of awareness and empathy in caregiving. Understanding these conditions allows us to provide better support and create a nurturing environment for our loved ones. Empathy fosters deeper connections and helps us navigate the inevitable changes with compassion and understanding.

In conclusion, the journey through Alzheimer's and dementia is undeniably challenging, but it is also a journey of love, resilience, and growth. By fostering awareness and empathy, we can honor the experiences of those affected and support each other through the ups and downs. As we listen to the stories of families like the Thompsons and Garcias, we are reminded that we are not alone in this journey. Together, we can create a compassionate community that uplifts and supports everyone touched by Alzheimer's and dementia.

Chapter 2
Understanding Alzheimer's and Dementia

Alzheimer's disease and dementia are terms that often come up in conversations about aging and cognitive health. While many people use these terms interchangeably, they refer to different concepts. This guide aims to clarify what Alzheimer's and dementia are, their differences, common risk factors, and how to recognize early signs and symptoms.

What is Dementia?

Dementia is not a specific disease but an umbrella term that describes a variety of symptoms affecting memory, thinking, and social abilities. It interferes with daily life and can impact a person's ability to perform everyday tasks. Dementia can occur due to several conditions, the most common being Alzheimer's disease.

Common Types of Dementia:

Alzheimer's disease: 60-80% of instances of dementia are caused by this disease. It mostly impacts cognitive function and memory. **Vascular Dementia:** Often caused by strokes or other blood flow issues in the brain, this type affects reasoning, planning, and judgment.

Lewy Body Dementia: Characterized by abnormal protein deposits in the brain, it affects memory, movement, and sleep.

Frontotemporal Dementia: This affects the front and sides of the brain and can lead to changes in personality and behavior.

What is Alzheimer's Disease?

Alzheimer's disease is a specific type of dementia that primarily impacts memory and cognitive abilities. Since the illness is progressive, symptoms progressively get worse over time. Cognitive loss is partly caused by the death and degradation of brain cells brought on by Alzheimer's disease.

Principal Aspects of Alzheimer's Disease:

One of the first and most obvious symptoms is memory loss.

Language issues include trouble following conversations or coming up with the appropriate words.

Disorientation is the state of not knowing where you are, when you are, or what to do.

Behavioral Modifications: Changes in mood, anxiety, or sadness.

Variations As opposed to dementia and Alzheimer's

Not all dementia is Alzheimer's, even though Alzheimer's is one kind of it.

Here are the key differences:

Aspect	Dementia	Alzheimer's Disease

Aspect	Dementia	Alzheimer's Disease
Definition	General term for decline in cognitive function	Specific type of dementia
Symptoms	Varies based on the type	Memory loss, language issues, disorientation
Progression	Can vary widely	Progressive, worsening over time
Cause	Multiple causes (e.g., strokes, injuries)	Unknown, but involves brain cell degeneration
Treatment	Depends on type and cause	Focuses on managing symptoms and slowing progression

Common Risk Factors for Alzheimer's and Dementia

Understanding the risk factors for Alzheimer's and dementia can help you or your loved ones take proactive steps toward brain health. Among the most prevalent risk factors are:

Age: The risk increases as individuals get older. Most people diagnosed with Alzheimer's are 65 or older.

Family History: A family history of Alzheimer's increases the risk, suggesting a genetic component.

Genetics: Certain genes, such as the APOE-e4 gene, are linked to a higher risk of Alzheimer's.

Cardiovascular Health: Risk factors for cardiovascular disease include diabetes, high blood pressure, and high cholesterol.

Lifestyle Factors: Lack of physical activity, poor diet, smoking, and excessive alcohol consumption can contribute to cognitive decline.

Head Injuries: Traumatic brain injuries may increase the risk of dementia later in life.

Recognizing Early Signs and Symptoms

Identifying early signs and symptoms of Alzheimer's and dementia can lead to earlier diagnosis and better management. Here are some typical indicators to look out for:

Memory Loss: Frequently forgetting recent events, important dates, or names.

Difficulty Completing Familiar Tasks: Struggling to perform routine activities, such as cooking a favorite recipe or managing finances.

Confusion About Time or Place: Losing track of dates, seasons, or where they are.

Challenges in Problem-Solving: Difficulty following a plan or working with numbers.

Changes in Mood or Personality: Experiencing mood swings, confusion, or anxiety.

Withdrawal from Social Activities: Steer clear of loved ones, friends, and past pursuits.

The Emotional Impact on Families

The journey through Alzheimer's and dementia affects not only the individuals diagnosed but also their families. Caregivers often face emotional challenges, including grief, frustration, and helplessness.

Tips for Families:

Educate Yourself: Understanding Alzheimer's and dementia helps families provide better support.

Communicate Openly: Encourage family members to share their feelings and concerns.

Seek Support: Consider joining support groups for caregivers to share experiences and strategies.

Conclusion

Understanding the differences between Alzheimer's and dementia is crucial for families and caregivers. By recognizing common risk factors and early signs, individuals can take steps to seek help and provide support. The emotional journey can be challenging, but knowledge and empathy can make a significant difference. As research continues, we hope for better treatments and support for those affected by these conditions.

Chapter 3
Diagnosis and Stages

Getting a diagnosis of Alzheimer's or another form of dementia can be a daunting experience. It often involves many steps, including medical evaluations, tests, and discussions with healthcare professionals. Understanding the diagnosis process and knowing what to expect at each stage can help alleviate some anxiety and uncertainty. This guide aims to provide a comprehensive overview of diagnosing Alzheimer's and dementia, with tips for navigating medical appointments and advocating for your loved one.

What is a Diagnosis?

A diagnosis is the process of determining the nature of a health issue based on signs, symptoms, and tests. In the case of Alzheimer's and dementia, a diagnosis can help identify the specific type of dementia and guide treatment and care decisions. While it can be emotional and overwhelming, a proper diagnosis can lead to better management of the condition.

The Importance of Early Diagnosis

Early diagnosis of Alzheimer's or dementia is crucial for several reasons:

Planning for the Future: Knowing the diagnosis allows families to plan for future care needs.

Access to Treatment: Early intervention can help manage symptoms and may improve quality of life.

Support and Resources: Families can access support services and resources sooner.

Involvement in Decision-Making: Patients may want to be involved in care decisions while they still have the capacity to express their wishes.

The Diagnosis Process

The diagnosis process for Alzheimer's and dementia typically involves several steps. Each stage may vary depending on individual circumstances, but the overall process generally follows these stages:

Initial Consultation

What to Expect: The process often begins with a visit to a primary care physician. During this visit, the doctor will ask questions about symptoms, medical history, and any changes in behavior or cognitive function.

Tips for Families: Prepare for this appointment by writing down specific examples of concerning behaviors or changes. Note when these changes began and how they affect daily life.

Physical Examination

What to Expect: The doctor will conduct a physical examination to rule out other health conditions that may cause similar symptoms. This may include checking vital signs, conducting neurological exams, and assessing overall health.

Tips for Families: Encourage your loved one to be honest about their symptoms during the examination. It may also be helpful to bring a list of current medications, as some medications can impact cognitive function.

Cognitive and Neuropsychological Tests

What to Expect: The doctor may administer cognitive tests to assess memory, problem-solving, attention, and language skills. These tests can vary in length and complexity but are designed to evaluate cognitive function.

Tips for Families: Remind your loved one that these tests are not pass/fail. They are tools for understanding their cognitive abilities. Providing reassurance can help reduce anxiety about testing.

Brain Imaging Tests

What to Expect: Depending on the results of the initial assessments, the doctor may order brain imaging tests, such as MRI or CT scans. These tests help identify changes in brain structure, rule out other conditions (like tumors or strokes), and assess the extent of any damage.

Tips for Families: Explain the imaging process to your loved one. Let them know that these tests are non-invasive and help provide a clearer picture of their brain health.

Laboratory Tests

What to Expect: Blood tests may be conducted to rule out other causes of cognitive decline, such as vitamin deficiencies, thyroid problems, or infections.

Tips for Families: Encourage your loved one to stay calm during blood tests. Remind them that these tests are routine and help doctors find the right diagnosis.

Referral to Specialists

What to Expect: If Alzheimer's or dementia is suspected, your loved one may be referred to a neurologist, geriatrician, or psychiatrist who specializes in cognitive disorders. These specialists may conduct further assessments and provide more specific diagnoses.

Tips for Families: It can be beneficial to accompany your loved one to these appointments. To make sure you comprehend the material given, make notes and ask questions.

Understanding the Diagnosis

Once all assessments and tests are complete, the healthcare team will review the results and determine a diagnosis. Here's what to expect:

Receiving the Diagnosis: The doctor will discuss the findings and explain the diagnosis, whether it's Alzheimer's, vascular dementia, or another form. This conversation may include details about what the diagnosis means for your loved one's health and cognitive function.

Discussing Next Steps: The doctor will outline possible treatment options, including medications and lifestyle changes that can help manage symptoms and improve quality of life.

Emotional Response: It's normal to experience a range of emotions upon receiving a diagnosis. Family members may feel grief, fear, or uncertainty about the future.

Navigating Medical Appointments

Medical appointments can be overwhelming, but there are ways to make the process smoother:

Prepare Ahead of Time: Before each appointment, review notes on symptoms, concerns, and questions. Bring along any necessary medical records or test results.

Pose inquiries: Inquire freely if you have any questions if something is unclear. Effective care requires that the patient understands the diagnosis, available treatments, and what to expect going forward.
Make a note of it: Make notes of all the pertinent information during the visit, such as the doctor's suggestions and treatment plans. This can come in handy down the road.

Engage Your loved one: Encourage the person you care about to take part in conversations on their health. It is important to take their preferences and point of view into account while making decisions.
Speaking Up for Your Special Someone
One of the most important aspects of the diagnostic and

care process is standing up for your loved one. The following are some tactics for successful advocacy:

Communicate Openly: Share any concerns you have about your loved one's health and well-being with their healthcare team. Don't hesitate to speak up if you feel something is not being addressed.

Stay Informed: Research Alzheimer's and dementia to better understand the conditions. Being knowledgeable will help you advocate for your loved one's needs.

Seek Support Services: Look for local support groups, resources, and organizations that can provide information and assistance. These can be invaluable for both caregivers and individuals living with dementia.

Consider Legal and Financial Planning: Discuss long-term care planning with your loved one. Consider working with an attorney to establish advanced directives, power of attorney, and other important documents.

Living with the Diagnosis

Once a diagnosis is made, it's essential to understand what to expect in the future. Alzheimer's and dementia are progressive conditions, meaning they will likely worsen over time. However, each individual's journey is unique. Here are some general stages to be aware of:

Early Stage: Individuals may still function independently but may experience mild cognitive changes. Memory lapses and difficulty concentrating may become noticeable.

Middle Stage: This stage often involves more pronounced memory loss, confusion about time and place, and changes in behavior or personality. People could require support with everyday tasks.

Late Stage: In the final stages, individuals may lose the ability to communicate, recognize loved ones, or perform basic self-care tasks. Care needs increase significantly during this stage.

Tips for Caregivers

Navigating the challenges of caregiving can be overwhelming. Here are some pointers to assist you with your journey:

Practice Self-Care: Caring for a loved one can be physically and emotionally draining. Prioritize your well-being by taking breaks, seeking support, and maintaining your health.

Maintain Routine: Establishing a daily routine can provide structure and comfort for your loved one. Familiar activities and schedules can help reduce confusion and anxiety.

Communicate with Compassion: Approach conversations with empathy and understanding. Simple, clear communication can help your loved one feel more at ease.

Engage in Activities: Encourage participation in activities that bring joy and stimulate cognitive function, such as puzzles, music, or arts and crafts.

Conclusion

The journey of diagnosing Alzheimer's and dementia can be challenging for individuals and families alike. By understanding the process and knowing what to expect at each stage, families can better navigate medical appointments and advocate for their loved ones. While the diagnosis may bring uncertainty and emotion, it also opens the door to understanding, support, and access to resources that can improve quality of life. By fostering a supportive and compassionate environment, families can help their loved ones live their best lives despite the challenges of Alzheimer's and dementia.

Chapter 4
Treatment and Care Options for Alzheimer's and Dementia

Caring for someone with Alzheimer's or dementia can feel overwhelming. However, understanding the treatment and care options available can empower caregivers to provide better support. This guide covers medications, therapies, daily care strategies, and practical tips for creating a supportive home environment.

Understanding Alzheimer's and Dementia Treatment Options

Alzheimer's and dementia care typically focuses on managing symptoms, enhancing quality of life, and ensuring safety. Treatment options include medications, various therapies, and practical strategies for daily living.

Medications for Alzheimer's and Dementia

Medications play a crucial role in managing symptoms and improving the quality of life for individuals with Alzheimer's and dementia. An overview of frequently prescribed drugs is provided below:

Cholinesterase Inhibitors

Purpose: These medications help improve communication between nerve cells by increasing levels of acetylcholine, a neurotransmitter.

Examples: Donepezil (Aricept), Rivastigmine (Exelon), and Galantamine (Razadyne).

Common Uses: They are often prescribed for mild to moderate Alzheimer's disease.

Possible Side Effects: Nausea, diarrhea, insomnia, muscle cramps, and fatigue.

Memantine

Purpose: Memantine helps regulate glutamate, another neurotransmitter involved in learning and memory.

Common Uses: This medication is typically prescribed for moderate to severe Alzheimer's disease.

Possible Side Effects: Dizziness, headache, confusion, and constipation.

Antidepressants

Purpose: Individuals with Alzheimer's or dementia may experience depression or anxiety. Antidepressants can help manage these symptoms.

Examples: Selective serotonin reuptake inhibitors (SSRIs) like sertraline (Zoloft) and citalopram (Celexa).

Common Uses: They are used for individuals experiencing mood disorders.

Possible Side Effects: Nausea, weight gain, fatigue, and sexual dysfunction.

Antipsychotic Medications

Purpose: These medications may be prescribed for behavioral symptoms such as agitation, aggression, or severe confusion.

Examples: Risperidone (Risperdal) and quetiapine (Seroquel).

Common Uses: Used with caution in Alzheimer's patients, as they can increase the risk of serious side effects.

Possible Side Effects: Sedation, weight gain, and increased risk of stroke.

Other Medications

Purpose: Various medications may be used to manage specific symptoms such as sleep disturbances or pain.

Examples: Sleep aids, anti-anxiety medications, and medications for pain management.

Common Uses: Based on individual needs and symptom presentation.

Possible Side Effects: Vary based on the specific medication.

Therapies for Alzheimer's and Dementia

In addition to medications, various therapies can enhance the quality of life for individuals with

Alzheimer's and dementia. These therapies focus on emotional, cognitive, and physical well-being.

Cognitive Stimulation Therapy (CST)

Purpose: CST involves engaging in activities that stimulate thinking, concentration, and memory.

Activities: Group sessions or individual activities such as puzzles, word games, and memory recall exercises.

Benefits: Helps maintain cognitive function and reduces feelings of isolation.

Reality Orientation Therapy

Purpose: This therapy aims to help individuals stay connected to their surroundings and improve awareness of time, place, and person.

Techniques: Providing regular reminders about time and place, using calendars, and discussing current events.

Benefits: Can reduce confusion and enhance overall well-being.

Reminiscence Therapy

Purpose: This approach encourages individuals to recall past experiences and memories.

Activities: Using photographs, music, or familiar objects to trigger memories.

Benefits: Promotes social interaction, reduces feelings of anxiety, and helps maintain identity.

Art and Music Therapy

Purpose: Creative expression through art and music can be therapeutic for individuals with dementia.

Activities: Engaging in painting, drawing, or listening to and playing music.

Benefits: Encourages emotional expression, improves mood, and stimulates memories.

Physical Therapy

Purpose: Maintaining physical health and mobility is essential for individuals with Alzheimer's and dementia.

Activities: Gentle exercises, walking, and balance training tailored to individual abilities.

Benefits: Improves physical health, enhances mobility, and promotes overall well-being.

Daily Care Strategies for Alzheimer's and Dementia

Daily care for individuals with Alzheimer's and dementia involves creating a structured, supportive environment. Here are practical strategies to implement:

Establish a Routine

Importance: Consistency helps individuals feel secure and reduces anxiety.

Implementation: Create a daily schedule that includes meal times, activities, and rest periods. Use visual schedules or calendars to provide reminders.

Simplify the Environment

Importance: Reducing clutter and distractions can help individuals focus and feel more at ease.

Implementation: Keep living spaces organized and remove unnecessary items. Label rooms and essential items (e.g., "Bathroom," "Kitchen") to aid navigation.

Communication Techniques

Importance: Clear communication is essential to avoid confusion and frustration.

Implementation: Use simple, direct language, and maintain eye contact. Be patient, listen actively, and give individuals time to respond.

Encourage Independence

Importance: Supporting individuals in maintaining independence fosters dignity and self-esteem.

Implementation: Offer choices in daily activities (e.g., what to wear, what to eat) and allow them to participate in simple tasks (e.g., setting the table).

Promote Social Interaction

Importance: Social engagement is vital for emotional well-being and cognitive stimulation.

Implementation: Encourage family visits, organize small gatherings, or participate in community activities. Engage in conversations and shared activities like games or puzzles.

Monitor Nutrition and Hydration

Importance: Proper nutrition and hydration are crucial for overall health.

Implementation: Offer balanced meals and snacks, and encourage regular water intake. Consider meal planning and preparation together to involve your loved one.

Ensure Safety

Importance: Safety is a top priority for individuals with cognitive impairments.

Implementation: Remove hazards, such as loose rugs or clutter, and install safety features (e.g., grab bars in bathrooms). Consider using GPS tracking devices if wandering is a concern.

Manage Behavioral Symptoms

Importance: Behavioral changes are common in individuals with dementia.

Implementation: Identify triggers for behaviors such as agitation or aggression, and respond calmly. Apply strategies for diverting their attention or shift their focus to another task.

Creating a Supportive Home Environment

Creating a nurturing home environment is key to enhancing the quality of life for individuals with Alzheimer's and dementia. Here are steps to create a supportive space:

Use Familiar Items

Purpose: Familiar items can provide comfort and trigger memories.

Implementation: Display photographs, personal belongings, and cherished objects throughout the home.

Optimize Lighting

Purpose: Proper lighting can reduce confusion and anxiety.

Implementation: Ensure spaces are well-lit and use natural light whenever possible. Avoid harsh lighting and minimize glare.

Incorporate Sensory Stimuli

Purpose: Engaging the senses can promote calm and connection.

Implementation: Use soft music, scented candles, or tactile items (e.g., blankets, fidget toys) to create a sensory-rich environment.

Designate Activity Areas

Purpose: Specific areas for activities can help structure daily routines.

Implementation: Set up spaces for reading, crafting, or watching movies. Make sure these spaces are welcoming and cozy.

Personalize Spaces

Purpose: Personal touches can create a sense of ownership and belonging.

Implementation: Involve your loved one in choosing decorations or arranging their space. Let them decide where to place items or furniture.

Provide Comfortable Seating

Purpose: Comfortable seating encourages relaxation and social interaction.

Implementation: Ensure chairs and couches are supportive and easily accessible. Consider using recliners or chairs with armrests for added comfort.

Conclusion

Caring for someone with Alzheimer's or dementia involves a combination of medical treatment, therapeutic approaches, and daily care strategies. Understanding these options empowers caregivers to provide effective support while maintaining the dignity and well-being of their loved ones. By creating a nurturing environment and implementing practical strategies, caregivers can significantly enhance the quality of life for individuals facing the challenges of Alzheimer's and dementia.

Caring for a loved one with these conditions is a journey that requires patience, empathy, and understanding. Remember, you are not alone in this experience. Seek support, gather resources, and continue to learn about the best ways to provide care. Every small step you take makes a difference in your loved one's life.

Chapter 5

Managing behavioral changes in individuals with Alzheimer's and dementia can be one of the most challenging aspects of caregiving. These changes can include aggression, agitation, wandering, and other behaviors that may be difficult to understand or address. Understanding why these behaviors occur and finding ways to respond effectively can help ease the stress on both the individual and their family.

Understanding Behavioral Changes in Alzheimer's and Dementia

Behavioral changes are common in individuals with Alzheimer's and other forms of dementia due to the progressive nature of these conditions, which affect the brain's ability to function. The changes in behavior are often a result of:

Cognitive Decline: As memory, judgment, and other cognitive abilities decline, the person may have trouble expressing themselves, leading to frustration and behavioral changes.

Emotional Distress: Feelings of confusion, fear, or insecurity may manifest in behaviors like aggression or withdrawal.

Physical Discomfort: Pain, hunger, fatigue, or other discomforts can trigger behaviors when the person is unable to communicate these needs effectively.

Environmental Triggers: A noisy room, unfamiliar surroundings, or even changes in routine can provoke reactions such as anxiety or agitation.

Common Behavioral Challenges and Effective Coping Strategies

1. Agitation and Aggression

Individuals with Alzheimer's and dementia may experience agitation, which can escalate into aggression. This can be triggered by confusion, frustration, fear, or physical discomfort.

Coping Strategies:

Identify Triggers: Try to observe what situations or factors seem to provoke agitation or aggression. It might be certain times of the day, specific tasks, or interactions with particular people.

Stay Calm: Respond in a calm, reassuring tone. Your demeanor can influence their emotions, so approach them with patience.

Redirect Attention: Distract the individual with a different activity or change the environment if possible. For instance, if they become upset while bathing, you can redirect their attention to music or a favorite picture.

Avoid Arguing: If they make statements that are not factual or express paranoid thoughts, avoid correcting them or arguing. Instead, validate their feelings and offer comfort.

Physical Contact: Sometimes, a gentle touch or holding their hand can calm agitation, but always approach slowly to avoid startling them.

2. Wandering

Wandering is a significant concern, as it can pose safety risks. It may be prompted by restlessness, disorientation, or a desire to go somewhere familiar.

Coping Strategies:

Provide Safe Areas for Walking: Create safe, enclosed areas where the person can walk freely. If this isn't possible, ensure doors are locked and have safety alarms installed.

Meet Their Needs: Make sure the person is not wandering because they are looking for something, such as the bathroom or food. Try to understand their routine to anticipate potential triggers.

Use Identification: If wandering becomes a regular issue, consider having the person wear an ID bracelet with their name and your contact information.

Utilize GPS Devices: Some devices can help track the individual's location, giving you peace of mind.

3. Sleep Disturbances

Sleep disturbances, such as difficulty falling asleep, staying asleep, or sundowning (increased confusion in the evening), are common.

Coping Strategies:

Establish a Bedtime Routine: Consistent routines help signal that it's time to wind down. This could include listening to calming music, dimming the lights, or reading a soothing book.

Limit Caffeine and Sugary Foods: Reducing these can improve sleep quality. Try offering a warm, caffeine-free drink before bed.

Encourage Daytime Activity: Help the individual engage in physical activity during the day to promote better sleep at night.

Keep the Bedroom Comfortable: Ensure the room is not too hot or cold and minimize noise and light to create a calm atmosphere.

4. Paranoia and Delusions

People with dementia may experience false beliefs or feelings of paranoia. For example, they may accuse others of stealing or think that people are spying on them.

Coping Strategies:

Avoid Confrontation: If they insist on their belief, avoid arguing. Instead, offer reassurances, distract with another activity, or acknowledge their feelings without confirming the belief.

Create a Safe Environment: Eliminate triggers that could fuel paranoia, such as unfamiliar items or noise.

Provide Reassurance: Frequently remind them that they are safe and loved. Sometimes, showing them familiar photos or objects can comfort them.

Supporting the Person and Their Family Emotionally

Behavioral changes can be emotionally distressing for both the individual and their family. Offering emotional support is essential for everyone involved.

1. Supporting the Individual

Practice Empathy: Try to see the world from their perspective. They may be experiencing confusion and fear, and responding with empathy can help them feel understood and cared for.

Stay Positive: Focus on what the individual can still do rather than what they've lost. Celebrating small achievements can boost their mood and confidence.

Foster Familiarity: Surround them with familiar objects, sounds, and routines to reduce anxiety. Consistent daily activities can bring comfort and stability.

Use Gentle Communication: Speak slowly, use simple words, and maintain eye contact. Avoid asking complex questions, and offer choices instead of open-ended prompts.

Music and Art Therapy: Engaging in creative activities can be a powerful way to connect emotionally and can also help manage behavioral symptoms.

2. Supporting Family Members

Encourage Open Communication: Family members should feel comfortable sharing their feelings and experiences. Open communication can reduce misunderstandings and foster mutual support.

Provide Education: Understanding Alzheimer's and dementia can help family members know what to expect and how to respond to various behaviors.

Establish Support Networks: Encourage family members to join support groups where they can connect with others facing similar experiences. This can offer both helpful guidance and emotional comfort.

Seek Professional Guidance: Sometimes, consulting a professional, such as a therapist or counselor, can help family members cope with the emotional strain.

3. Self-Care for Caregivers

Take Breaks: Regularly taking time off to recharge is vital for caregivers. Short breaks can provide the mental

reset needed to return to caregiving with renewed patience.
Ask for Help: Reach out to other family members, friends, or professional services to share the load. Caregiving can be overwhelming, and it's okay to seek assistance.
Practice Mindfulness or Meditation: Techniques such as meditation, yoga, or deep breathing can help caregivers manage stress.
Set Boundaries: Know your limits and don't hesitate to set boundaries regarding the care tasks you can handle.

Creating a Supportive Environment

The right environment can help reduce challenging behaviors and provide a sense of safety for the individual.
Maintain Consistency: Keep daily routines and surroundings as consistent as possible.
Simplify the Space: Reduce clutter and unnecessary stimuli that could overwhelm the person.
Use Visual Cues: Signs, labels, and familiar objects can help orient the individual and make navigation easier.
Limit Noise: Minimize loud or sudden sounds that can cause agitation.
Ensure Safety: Remove hazards such as loose rugs or sharp objects and secure potentially dangerous areas, like the kitchen.

Engaging in Activities

Meaningful activities can reduce feelings of boredom and restlessness, and help manage behaviors.

Tailor Activities to Their Abilities: Choose activities they can do and enjoy, whether it's simple crafts, gardening, or listening to music.
Encourage Physical Activity: Gentle exercise like walking or stretching can improve mood and reduce agitation.
Involve Them in Daily Tasks: Allow them to help with household chores to the extent they can manage, such as folding towels or setting the table.

The Power of Empathy and Patience

Managing behavioral changes in Alzheimer's and dementia requires a compassionate approach. Caregivers and family members should focus on the individual's emotions rather than the behavior itself. Understanding that these behaviors stem from changes in the brain can help foster a patient and loving attitude. Caregiving for a person with Alzheimer's is a journey of learning and adapting. Families should remind themselves that it's okay to seek help, take breaks, and acknowledge the challenges. By employing coping strategies and prioritizing emotional support, it's possible to create a supportive and understanding environment that benefits everyone involved.

Chapter 6
The Role of Diet in Managing Alzheimer's and Dementia

Nutrition plays a vital role in maintaining overall health, especially for individuals with Alzheimer's and dementia. A healthy diet can help support brain function, manage symptoms, and enhance overall well-being. This guide explores foods that promote brain health, offers meal planning ideas, and provides tips for encouraging healthy eating habits.

Understanding the Connection Between Diet and Brain Health

Research indicates that certain dietary patterns can influence brain health and cognitive function. A balanced diet rich in nutrients can help protect the brain from damage, support cognitive performance, and potentially slow the progression of Alzheimer's and dementia.

Important Nutritional Components for Brain Function:

Antioxidants: Assist in preventing the harm that oxidative stress causes to brain cells. present in vegetables and fruits.
Omega-3 Fatty Acids: May lower inflammation and are vital for brain function. present in walnuts, flaxseeds, and fatty fish.
B vitamins are essential for energy metabolism and brain

function. present in dairy products, leafy vegetables, and whole grains.

Polyphenols: May lessen the chance of cognitive decline and enhance brain function. present in green tea, dark chocolate, and berries.

Foods that Support Healthy Brain Function

A diet that includes particular foods can promote general wellbeing and brain health. Here are some important dietary types and ideas to think about:

Fruits and Vegetables

Berries: Blueberries, strawberries, and blackberries are rich in antioxidants and may enhance memory.

Leafy Greens: Spinach, kale, and broccoli are packed with vitamins and minerals that support brain health.

Cruciferous Vegetables: Cauliflower and Brussels sprouts contain compounds that may help protect brain cells.

Whole Grains

Examples: Brown rice, quinoa, whole wheat bread, and oatmeal.

Benefits: Provide energy and essential nutrients that support brain function.

Healthy Fats

Olive Oil: A primary source of healthy monounsaturated fats that promote heart and brain health.

Fatty Fish: Salmon, mackerel, and sardines are high in omega-3 fatty acids, which are beneficial for brain health.

Nuts and Seeds: Walnuts, almonds, chia seeds, and flaxseeds are excellent sources of healthy fats and nutrients.

Lean Proteins

Examples: Chicken, turkey, beans, lentils, and tofu.

Benefits: Provide essential amino acids that support brain health and overall functioning.

Dairy Products

Examples: Low-fat yogurt, milk, and cheese.

Benefits: Offer calcium, protein, and B vitamins that are important for brain health.

Herbs and Spices

Turmeric: Curcumin, an anti-inflammatory compound found in turmeric, may help with cognitive function.

Ginger: May lessen inflammation and enhance blood flow.

Ideas for Meal Planning

It can be easy and fun to design a diet plan that emphasizes foods that are good for the brain. Here are some suggestions to get you going:

Breakfast Ideas

Oatmeal with Berries: Cook oatmeal and top with fresh or frozen berries and a sprinkle of nuts.

Greek Yogurt Parfait: Layer Greek yogurt with mixed berries and a drizzle of honey, topped with granola.

Smoothie: Blend spinach, banana, almond milk, and a tablespoon of peanut butter for a nutritious start to the day.

Lunch Ideas

Quinoa Salad: Combine cooked quinoa, diced vegetables (like bell peppers and cucumber), and a dressing of olive oil and lemon juice.

Whole Grain Wrap: Fill a whole-grain wrap with lean turkey, leafy greens, and avocado. Serve with a side of baby carrots.

Vegetable Soup: Make a hearty soup using low-sodium broth, mixed vegetables, and beans.

Dinner Ideas

Grilled Salmon: Serve grilled salmon with steamed broccoli and quinoa.

Stir-Fried Vegetables: Sauté a mix of colorful vegetables with tofu or chicken, served over brown rice.

Lentil Curry: Prepare a lentil curry with spices, tomatoes, and spinach, served with brown rice or whole-grain naan.

Snack Ideas

Nut Mix: Create a mix of almonds, walnuts, and dried fruit for a quick snack.

Hummus & Veggies: Arrange bell peppers, carrots, and celery slices alongside hummus.

Apple Slices with Nut Butter: Slice apples and serve with almond or peanut butter for added protein.

Tips for Encouraging Healthy Eating Habits

Encouraging healthy eating habits can be challenging, especially for individuals with Alzheimer's and dementia. Here are some practical tips to promote nutritious eating:

Make Mealtime Enjoyable

Create a pleasant dining atmosphere with soft music, comfortable seating, and good lighting.

Encourage social interactions by eating together with family or friends.

Simplify Choices

Provide a limited selection of food options to reduce overwhelm.

Use colorful plates and utensils to make meals visually appealing.

Focus on Texture and Flavor

Prepare foods with a variety of textures and flavors to enhance the eating experience.

Experiment with different herbs and spices to add flavor without excess salt or sugar.

Incorporate Familiar Foods

Offer favorite foods and family recipes to promote a sense of comfort and familiarity.

Experiment with different herbs and spices to add flavor without excess salt or sugar.
Incorporate Familiar Foods
Offer favorite foods and family recipes to promote a sense of comfort and familiarity.
Encourage the individual to participate in meal planning and preparation.
Stay Hydrated
Encourage regular fluid intake by offering water, herbal teas, or flavored water.
Offer hydrating foods such as watermelon, cucumbers, and soups.
Monitor Portions
Serve smaller portions to avoid overwhelming the individual and allow for second servings if desired.
Use smaller plates and bowls to help with portion control.

Adapt to Individual Needs
Be mindful of any dietary restrictions or preferences.

Modify food textures if necessary (e.g., pureeing foods or cutting them into smaller pieces).

Creating a Brain-Healthy Meal Plan

Here's a sample meal plan for a week that incorporates brain-healthy foods:

Day 1:

Breakfast: Oatmeal with sliced bananas and walnuts.

Lunch : a salad of quinoa dressed with cucumber, cherry tomatoes, and olive oil.

Dinner: steamed broccoli, roasted sweet potatoes, and grilled chicken.

Day 2: Almond milk, spinach, and banana smoothie for breakfast.

Lunch: a turkey, lettuce, and avocado whole-grain wrap.

Dinner: asparagus and brown rice with baked fish.

Day 3: Greek yogurt with honey and mixed berries for breakfast.

Lunch would be whole-grain bread and lentil soup.

Supper is quinoa topped with stir-fried tofu and mixed veggies.

Day 4: Whole-grain bread and scrambled eggs with spinach for breakfast.

Lunch is a vinaigrette-dressed vegetable salad with chickpeas.

Dinner is black bean and corn chili made with turkey.

Day 5: Oatmeal with chia seeds and fresh fruit for breakfast.

Lunch: Hummus with carrot sticks and whole-grain crackers.

Dinner: Grilled shrimp with vegetable stir-fry and brown rice.

Day 6:

Breakfast: Cottage cheese with pineapple and almonds.

Lunch: Spinach salad with grilled chicken and balsamic dressing.

Dinner: Baked tilapia with quinoa and roasted Brussels sprouts.

Day 7:

Breakfast: Whole-grain pancakes topped with fresh strawberries.

Lunch: Stuffed bell peppers with brown rice and beans.

Dinner: Veggie curry with lentils served with whole-grain naan.

Conclusion

A well-balanced diet rich in brain-healthy foods can play a significant role in managing Alzheimer's and dementia. By incorporating fruits, vegetables, whole grains, healthy fats, lean proteins, and dairy products, caregivers can help support cognitive function and enhance overall well-being.

Meal planning ideas and practical tips for encouraging healthy eating habits can make a positive difference in the lives of individuals with these conditions. Remember, the journey of caregiving is about finding joy in everyday moments and making the most of each day. Every small change in diet and nutrition can lead to improved health and a better quality of life.

Chapter 7
Support for Families and Caregivers

Caring for someone with Alzheimer's or dementia can be both rewarding and challenging. Families and caregivers play a crucial role in supporting their loved ones, but it is essential to prioritize self-care and seek support along the way. This guide provides coping strategies, resources, and self-care tips, along with personal stories that highlight the importance of community and support in this journey.

Understanding the Role of Caregivers

Caregivers for individuals with Alzheimer's and dementia often find themselves in demanding and emotional roles. You may be a spouse, child, or friend, and the responsibilities can feel overwhelming at times. Recognizing the significance of your role and the challenges you face is the first step toward effective caregiving.

Key Responsibilities of Caregivers:

Daily Assistance: Helping with activities of daily living (ADLs) such as bathing, dressing, and eating.

Medication Management: Ensuring medications are taken as prescribed and managing any side effects.

Emotional Support: Providing comfort and understanding as cognitive abilities decline.

Communication: Adapting to changes in communication and finding new ways to connect.

Coping Strategies for Caregivers

Caring for someone with Alzheimer's or dementia can bring a range of emotions, from love and compassion to frustration and sadness. Here are some coping strategies to help you manage these feelings and maintain your well-being:

Educate Yourself

Understanding Alzheimer's and dementia helps you anticipate changes and challenges. Having knowledge can help you make wise judgments.

Personal Story: Mirabel, a caregiver for her mother with Alzheimer's, found comfort in reading books and attending workshops. She learned how to handle difficult behaviors and felt more prepared for the journey ahead.

Establish a Routine

Creating a consistent daily routine can provide structure and predictability, benefiting both you and your loved one.

People with dementia may experience less anxiety and bewilderment when they follow a routine.

Practice Patience

It's natural to feel frustrated when communicating or assisting your loved one. Practice patience and remind yourself that these changes are due to the disease, not their personality.

Personal Story: John learned to take deep breaths and count to ten when his wife struggled to remember simple things. This practice helped him respond calmly instead of reacting with frustration.

Seek Support

Making connections with others who are sympathetic to your circumstances can be quite helpful. Online and in-person support groups provide a secure environment for people to discuss their struggles, victories, and experiences.

Resource: The Alzheimer's Association offers local and virtual support groups for caregivers.

Set Boundaries

Understand your limits and know when to ask for help. It's okay to say no to additional responsibilities if you feel overwhelmed.

Setting boundaries helps you prioritize your well-being and provides time for self-care.

Practice Mindfulness

Engaging in mindfulness practices can help you stay grounded during stressful moments. Activities like deep breathing, meditation, or gentle yoga can enhance your emotional resilience.

Personal Story: Maria found that taking a few minutes each day for meditation helped her feel more centered and better equipped to handle her mother's changing moods.

Resources for Caregivers

Utilizing available resources can make a significant difference in your caregiving experience. Here are some worthwhile sites to think about:

Alzheimer's Association: Offers a wealth of information on Alzheimer's and dementia, including caregiver support, educational materials, and local resources.

Local Community Services: Many communities have services for seniors and caregivers, including adult day programs, respite care, and support groups.

Online Forums and Social Media Groups: Connecting with others online can provide additional support and insights from people experiencing similar challenges.

Caregiver Training Programs: Consider enrolling in training programs that provide practical skills and knowledge for managing care.

Self-Care Tips for Caregivers

Taking care of yourself is not just important; it is essential for your ability to care for others. Here are self-care tips to help you maintain your health and well-being:

Prioritize Your Health

Make time for regular check-ups, exercise, and healthy eating. Your physical health is crucial for managing stress and staying energized.

Engage in Hobbies

Dedicate time to activities that bring you joy. Whether it's gardening, painting, or reading, hobbies can provide a much-needed break from caregiving responsibilities.

Stay Connected

Maintain connections with friends and family. Social interactions can uplift your spirits and reduce feelings of isolation.

Ask for Help

Don't hesitate to reach out for help when needed. Whether it's asking a family member to lend a hand or hiring professional respite care, seeking support is a sign of strength, not weakness.

Take Breaks

Allow yourself short breaks throughout the day. Step outside for fresh air, enjoy a cup of tea, or take a short walk to recharge your mind.

Consider Respite Care

Respite care services provide temporary relief for caregivers. This can allow you to take time off to rest or attend to personal matters.

Personal Stories of Community and Support

Theodore's Story

Theodore cared for his father, who was diagnosed with Alzheimer's. Feeling overwhelmed, he joined a local support group. Sharing his experiences with others facing similar challenges brought him comfort. He learned new coping strategies and realized he wasn't alone in this journey.

Angela's Journey

Angela, a mother of two, was balancing her family life while caring for her grandmother with dementia. She discovered a local adult day program where her grandmother could engage in activities. This not only provided her grandmother with social interaction but also gave Angela precious time to focus on her children and herself.

Tom's Turning Point

Tom was hesitant to reach out for help until he realized how much caregiving was affecting his mental health. He began attending a support group, where he met others who understood his struggles. The friendships he formed became a vital source of support, helping him navigate the ups and downs of caregiving.

The Importance of Community

Building a community of support is vital for caregivers. You are not alone in this journey, and many individuals and organizations are ready to help. Reach out to family, friends, and community resources for assistance and encouragement. Creating a support network allows caregivers to share their feelings, seek advice, and celebrate their successes.

Conclusion

Caring for someone with Alzheimer's or dementia can be a profound journey filled with challenges and rewards. By implementing coping strategies, utilizing resources, and prioritizing self-care, you can navigate this path with resilience and compassion. Remember, you are not alone; support is available, and building connections can make a significant difference in your experience.

As you care for your loved one, take time to care for yourself. Every small step you take to support your well-being will enable you to provide better care and create meaningful moments with your loved one. Together, we can build a compassionate community that uplifts and supports caregivers and individuals living with Alzheimer's and dementia.

Chapter 8
A Comprehensive Collection of Expert Insights and Real-Life Stories on Alzheimer's and Dementia

Alzheimer's and dementia affect millions of individuals and their families worldwide. As these conditions progress, they bring challenges that can feel overwhelming. However, through expert insights and real-life stories, we can learn valuable lessons, gather advice, and find comfort in shared experiences. This narrative aims to engage readers by presenting diverse perspectives that enhance understanding and foster empathy.

Lessons Learned from Experts

Experts in the field of Alzheimer's and dementia offer valuable insights that can guide caregivers and families. Here are some key lessons drawn from their experiences:

1. The Importance of Early Detection

Dr. Bella Williams, a neurologist specializing in Alzheimer's disease, emphasizes the significance of early detection. "More effective management of the condition can result from early identification of Alzheimer's signs," she says.

Insight: Early diagnosis allows for better planning and access to resources that can help individuals and families prepare for the journey ahead.

Example: A patient named Robert was diagnosed at an early stage after his wife noticed changes in his memory. With support from healthcare professionals, they developed a care plan that included medication, regular check-ups, and activities to stimulate his mind.

2. Embracing Compassionate Communication

Dr. Elizabeth Chen, a geriatrician, stresses the importance of communication techniques tailored to those with Alzheimer's. She says, "You can greatly improve the interaction by using simple language, maintaining eye contact, and being patient."

Insight: Compassionate communication fosters connection, reducing frustration for both the caregiver and the person with dementia.

Example: Jenny, a caregiver for her mother with Alzheimer's, learned to speak slowly and clearly. She noticed that using pictures or gestures helped her mother understand better and engage in conversations.

3. The Role of Nutrition and Exercise

Nutrition and physical activity play critical roles in brain health. Dr. Hart Patel, a dietitian specializing in dementia care, notes, "A balanced diet rich in antioxidants, healthy fats, and lean proteins can help support brain function."

Insight: Incorporating regular physical activity can also slow cognitive decline and enhance overall well-being.

Example: Ellen, a daughter caring for her father, introduced him to a Mediterranean diet filled with fruits, vegetables, whole grains, and fish. Together, they went for daily walks, which not only improved his mood but also strengthened their bond.

4. The Value of Respite Care

Dr. Lisa Carter, a social worker specializing in caregiver support, emphasizes the necessity of respite care for caregivers. "Taking breaks is crucial for your mental and physical health. Caregivers often neglect their needs while focusing on their loved ones."

Insight: Respite care provides temporary relief, allowing caregivers to recharge and prevent burnout.

Example: Mark, a husband caring for his wife with dementia, felt exhausted and overwhelmed. He decided to explore respite care options, which allowed him to take weekend breaks. During this time, he reconnected with friends and engaged in hobbies he had set aside.

Real-Life Stories of Resilience

Stories of individuals and families navigating the complexities of Alzheimer's and dementia illustrate the emotional journey and the lessons learned along the way.

1. Sarah's Journey of Acceptance

Sarah, a 58-year-old woman, shares her experience caring for her husband, Tom, who was diagnosed with Alzheimer's at 60. At first, Sarah struggled with accepting the diagnosis. "I kept hoping it was a mistake," she recalls.

As the disease progressed, she learned to embrace the changes in Tom. "I came to understand that my responsibility was to encourage him and enjoy our time together," she says.

Lesson: Acceptance of the diagnosis allowed Sarah to focus on creating meaningful moments with Tom, such as listening to music, watching their favorite movies, and reminiscing about their life together.

2. Kevin's Perspective on Patience

Kevin is a caregiver for his mother, who has vascular dementia. Initially, he felt frustrated when she struggled to remember simple things. "I often raised my voice or reacted harshly," he admits.

After attending a caregiver support group, Kevin learned about the importance of patience. .. He says, "I began to realize that it was the illness, not her."

Lesson: Kevin's journey highlights the need for caregivers to practice patience and empathy, which can significantly improve the relationship and enhance the quality of care.

3. Angel's Advocacy for Awareness

Angel's father was diagnosed with Alzheimer's, and she quickly became an advocate for awareness. "I realized how little people understood about this disease, and I wanted to change that," she shares.

Angel organized community events to educate others about Alzheimer's and dementia. She invited speakers, held workshops, and created informational materials to distribute. "Raising awareness helped not only my family but others in our community," she explains.

Lesson: Advocacy can empower caregivers and families, fostering understanding and support for those affected by Alzheimer's and dementia.

4. Tom's Journey of Rediscovery

Tom, a retired teacher, faced his diagnosis of Alzheimer's with courage. Instead of retreating from life, he embraced new experiences. He started attending art classes, exploring his creativity, and connecting with fellow artists.

"Art became my therapy," he says. ""I found that painting was a joyful and satisfying way for me to express myself.

Lesson: Engaging in creative outlets can provide individuals with Alzheimer's an opportunity for self-expression and fulfillment, fostering a sense of identity despite cognitive decline.

5. Matilda's Story of Resilience

Matilda, a young woman, found herself caring for her grandmother with dementia after her mother passed away. The weight of responsibility felt heavy, but Emily discovered strength within herself she didn't know existed.

"I learned to take it one day at a time," she reflects. "There were days when I felt overwhelmed, but I reached out to friends and family for support."

Lesson: Building a support network is essential for caregivers, providing emotional relief and practical assistance during challenging times.

Expert Insights on Coping Strategies

Experts offer additional strategies for coping with the challenges of caregiving and enhancing the quality of life for both caregivers and individuals with dementia.

1. Mindfulness Practices

Dr. Rebecca Adams, a psychologist specializing in caregiver stress, recommends mindfulness practices. "Mindfulness can help caregivers stay present and reduce anxiety," she explains.

Insight: Techniques such as deep breathing, meditation, and yoga can promote relaxation and emotional balance.

Example: Lisa, a caregiver for her husband, started a daily meditation practice. "It helped me manage stress and approach caregiving with a clearer mind," she shares.

2. Engaging in Support Groups

Participating in support groups is a powerful way for caregivers to share their experiences. Dr. Michael Turner, a geriatric psychiatrist, emphasizes the value of these gatherings. "Connecting with others who understand your struggles can provide validation and new perspectives."

Insight: Support groups can foster a sense of community and reduce feelings of isolation.

Example: Nancy joined a support group for caregivers of individuals with Alzheimer's. "Hearing others' stories made me feel less alone," she says. "It was comforting to know that we were all in this together."

3. Creating a Safe Environment

Dr. Jennifer Hill, an occupational therapist, stresses the importance of creating a safe home environment for individuals with dementia. "Making small adjustments can significantly enhance their safety and comfort," she explains.

Insight: Simple changes like removing tripping hazards, labeling doors, and using night lights can prevent accidents.

Example: Kevin modified his home to ensure it was safe for his mother, reducing her anxiety and enhancing her independence.

The Importance of Self-Care

Self-care is crucial for caregivers, as it allows them to recharge and maintain their physical and mental health. Here are some self-care strategies shared by experts and caregivers:

1. Prioritizing Personal Time

Dr. Laura Simmons, a clinical psychologist, emphasizes the necessity of taking personal time. "Caregivers often neglect their own needs, which can lead to burnout," she warns.

Insight: Carving out time for yourself, even for short periods, is essential for maintaining balance.

Example: Mark began scheduling weekly outings with friends to enjoy activities he loved. "It reminded me of who I was outside of caregiving," he shares.

2. Finding Joy in Simple Moments

Finding joy in everyday moments can help caregivers stay grounded. Dr. Angela Ramirez, a family therapist, encourages caregivers to appreciate small victories. "No matter how small the good days are, celebrate them," she says.

Insight: Focusing on positive experiences can improve emotional well-being.

Example: Jenny started keeping a gratitude journal, jotting down moments of joy with her mother. "It shifted my perspective and reminded me of the beauty in our time together," she says.

Implication: Guardianship gives a designated person the legal authority to make decisions for someone deemed incapacitated.

Practical Tip: Consider legal advice early to understand the guardianship process and implications.

Financial Considerations

Financial planning is critical for families managing Alzheimer's and dementia, as care costs can escalate quickly. Here are important financial considerations:

1. Understand the Costs of Care

The costs of care can vary widely based on the stage of dementia, care settings, and geographic location. Key areas of expense may include:

- **In-home care** Hiring caretakers to help with daily tasks is known as in-home care.

- **Adult day programs:** Providing social interaction and activities during the day.
- **Assisted living or nursing homes:** Long-term care facilities for individuals with higher needs.

Practical Tip: Research local care options and associated costs to prepare a realistic budget.

2. Evaluate Insurance Options

Explore various insurance policies that may help cover costs:

The Importance of Self-Care

Self-care is crucial for caregivers, as it allows them to recharge and maintain their physical and mental health. Here are some self-care strategies shared by experts and caregivers:

1. Prioritizing Personal Time

Dr. Laura Simmons, a clinical psychologist, emphasizes the necessity of taking personal time. "Caregivers often neglect their own needs, which can lead to burnout," she warns.

Insight: Carving out time for yourself, even for short periods, is essential for maintaining balance.

Example: Mark began scheduling weekly outings with friends to enjoy activities he loved. "It reminded me of who I was outside of caregiving," he shares.

2. Finding Joy in Simple Moments

Finding joy in everyday moments can help caregivers stay grounded. Dr. Angela Ramirez, a family therapist, encourages caregivers to appreciate small victories. "No matter how small the good days are, celebrate them," she says.

Insight: Focusing on positive experiences can improve emotional well-being.

Example: Jenny started keeping a gratitude journal, jotting down moments of joy with her mother. "It shifted my perspective and reminded me of the beauty in our time together," she says.

3. Connecting with Nature

Research shows that spending time in nature can reduce stress and enhance well-being. Dr. Oliver Hayes, an environmental psychologist, notes, "Nature has a calming effect on the mind and body."

Insight: Regular walks in nature can provide caregivers with a refreshing escape.

Example: Emily found solace in local parks, taking her grandmother for walks. "The verdancy and clean air lifted our spirits," she says.

Conclusion

The journey through Alzheimer's and dementia is filled with challenges, but it also presents opportunities for growth, connection, and resilience. By gathering expert insights and real-life stories, we can better understand the experiences of those affected by these conditions.

From early detection and compassionate communication to the importance of self-care and advocacy, the lessons learned resonate deeply. Each story shared reflects the strength of individuals and families navigating this complex landscape.

As we embrace these insights and experiences, may we foster compassion, awareness, and support for all those touched by Alzheimer's and dementia. Together, we can create a community that uplifts and empowers, ensuring that no one faces this journey alone.

Chapter 9
Planning for the Future

As Alzheimer's and dementia progress, it becomes increasingly important for individuals and families to plan for the future. Planning can provide peace of mind and help ensure that wishes are respected. This guide will cover legal, financial, and end-of-life considerations for families dealing with these conditions, along with practical tips to navigate these complex topics.

Understanding the Importance of Planning

Planning for the future is crucial for anyone facing a diagnosis of Alzheimer's or dementia. Here are some key reasons why:

- **Ensures Wishes Are Respected:** Proper planning helps ensure that a person's preferences regarding care and financial decisions are honored.
- **Reduces Stress for Family:** Having plans in place alleviates stress and confusion for family members who may need to make decisions on behalf of their loved ones.
- **Provides Financial Security:** Early planning can help manage the costs associated with care, reducing the financial burden on families.

Planning is best approached early in the diagnosis. The sooner decisions are made, the more control individuals can retain over their future.

Legal Considerations

Legal considerations are essential for individuals with Alzheimer's and dementia to ensure that their wishes are honored and their rights are protected. Here are the key legal documents to consider:

1. Power of Attorney (POA)

A Power of Attorney (POA) is a legal document that designates someone to make financial and legal decisions on behalf of an individual. This can involve processing investments, paying payments, and maintaining financial accounts.

- **Types of POA:**
    - **General POA:** Grants broad powers to the designated person.
    - **Durable POA:** Remains in effect even if the person becomes incapacitated.

Practical Tip: Choose someone trustworthy and capable, and discuss your wishes with them beforehand.

2. Healthcare Proxy

A healthcare proxy (or medical power of attorney) designates someone to make healthcare decisions if the individual becomes unable to do so. This includes choices about treatments, medications, and end-of-life care.

- **Considerations:**
    - Discuss specific healthcare preferences with the appointed proxy.
    - Ensure the proxy understands your values and wishes regarding medical care.

Practical Tip: Review the proxy designation regularly, especially as circumstances change.

3. Living Will

A living will is a legal document that outlines an individual's preferences for medical treatment in specific situations, particularly in end-of-life scenarios.

- **Key Aspects:**
    - Preferences regarding life-sustaining treatments.
    - Wishes about pain management and comfort care.

Practical Tip: Be clear and specific in your living will to avoid confusion later.

4. Guardianship

If an individual with dementia has not designated a POA or healthcare proxy, a family member may need to pursue guardianship through the court. This legal procedure may be expensive and time-consuming.

Implication: Guardianship gives a designated person the legal authority to make decisions for someone deemed incapacitated.

Practical Tip: Consider legal advice early to understand the guardianship process and implications.

Financial Considerations

Financial planning is critical for families managing Alzheimer's and dementia, as care costs can escalate quickly. Here are important financial considerations:

1. Understand the Costs of Care

The costs of care can vary widely based on the stage of dementia, care settings, and geographic location. Key areas of expense may include:

- **In-home care** Hiring caretakers to help with daily tasks is known as in-home care.
- **Adult day programs**: Providing social interaction and activities during the day.
- **Assisted living or nursing homes**: Long-term care facilities for individuals with higher needs.

Practical Tip: Research local care options and associated costs to prepare a realistic budget.

2. Evaluate Insurance Options

Explore various insurance policies that may help cover costs:

- **Health Insurance:** Understand what your health insurance plan covers regarding Alzheimer's and dementia care.
- **Long-Term Care Insurance:** Consider policies that specifically cover long-term care services.

Practical Tip: Review policy details and exclusions carefully to avoid surprises later.

3. Medicaid and Medicare

Familiarize yourself with the eligibility criteria and coverage options for Medicaid and Medicare. These programs can help offset costs for qualified individuals.

- **Medicaid:** Provides assistance to low-income individuals and may cover long-term care costs.
- **Medicare:** Offers limited coverage for skilled nursing facilities and certain home health services.

Practical Tip: Apply for Medicaid well before the need arises, as the process can take time.

4. Create a Financial Plan

Creating a comprehensive financial plan can help manage resources effectively. Consider:

- **Budgeting:** Track monthly expenses related to care.
- **Asset Management:** Decide how to manage assets to qualify for Medicaid if necessary.

- **Savings:** Set aside funds specifically for future care needs.

Practical Tip: Consult a financial planner experienced in elder care to help navigate these decisions.

End-of-Life Considerations

End-of-life planning is a sensitive but necessary part of the process. Addressing these issues early can reduce anxiety and uncertainty for both individuals and their families.

1. Discuss End-of-Life Wishes

It is crucial to have open conversations about end-of-life wishes with family members. Discuss topics such as:

- **Preferred place of care:** Whether to stay at home or move to a facility.
- **Resuscitation preferences:** Whether to pursue resuscitation efforts or allow a natural death.

Practical Tip: Use clear and compassionate language during these discussions to ensure understanding.

2. Funeral and Burial Arrangements

Planning for funeral and burial arrangements in advance can ease the burden on family members later. Consider discussing:

- **Type of service:** Traditional burial, cremation, or other options.

- **Financial arrangements:** Prepaying for services or setting aside funds.

Practical Tip: Document your wishes and share them with family members to avoid confusion later.

3. Hospice Care

Hospice care focuses on comfort and quality of life during the end-of-life stage. It is important to consider:

- **When to start hospice:** Typically when the individual is no longer seeking curative treatments.
- **Services provided:** Pain management, emotional support, and assistance for caregivers.

Practical Tip: Research local hospice providers early and discuss options with healthcare providers.

Navigating Complex Topics

Navigating the legal, financial, and end-of-life considerations can feel overwhelming. Here are practical tips for families:

1. Start Early

Begin planning as soon as a diagnosis is made. This approach allows for more thoughtful decisions and ensures that individuals retain control over their choices.

2. Involve the Entire Family

Engage family members in discussions and decisions. This collaboration fosters understanding and support among all involved.

3. Seek Professional Guidance

Consult professionals, such as elder law attorneys, financial planners, and healthcare providers, to guide you through the complexities of planning.

4. Keep Documentation Organized

Maintain all legal and financial documents in a secure and organized location. Create a folder or digital file that is easily accessible to family members.

5. Regularly Review Plans

Review and update legal and financial plans regularly, especially as circumstances change. This ensures that all documents reflect current wishes and conditions.

Conclusion

Planning for the future in the context of Alzheimer's and dementia is vital for ensuring that wishes are respected and families feel supported. By addressing legal, financial, and end-of-life considerations early, families can navigate these complex topics with confidence and clarity.

Through open communication, thorough planning, and seeking professional guidance, families can create a roadmap that honors the dignity of their loved ones while alleviating stress and uncertainty for themselves.

Remember, planning is not just about preparing for the worst; it's about fostering peace of mind and preserving the quality of life throughout the journey.

Chapter 10
Conclusion to the Guide on Alzheimer's and Dementia

The journey through Alzheimer's and dementia is profound and complex, affecting not only the individuals diagnosed but also their families and caregivers. This guide has explored various aspects of navigating these conditions, from understanding the differences between Alzheimer's and other forms of dementia to planning for the future. As we conclude, let's summarize the key takeaways and offer additional resources for support and information.

Key Takeaways

1. Understanding Alzheimer's and Dementia

Definitions: Alzheimer's is a specific type of dementia that affects memory, thinking, and behavior. Dementia is an umbrella term for a range of cognitive impairments that interfere with daily life.

Differences: While all Alzheimer's is dementia, not all dementia is Alzheimer's. It is essential to comprehend these differences in order to manage effectively.

2. Recognizing Early Signs and Symptoms

Common Symptoms: Early signs may include memory loss, difficulty completing familiar tasks, and challenges in planning or problem-solving Early detection of these symptoms can facilitate prompt diagnosis and treatment.

Importance of Awareness: Awareness of these symptoms helps in seeking medical advice promptly, which can improve the quality of care.

3. Legal and Financial Planning

Power of Attorney and Healthcare Proxy: Designating trusted individuals to make financial and healthcare decisions ensures that your wishes are respected.

Financial Considerations: Understanding costs associated with care and exploring insurance options can alleviate financial stress.

4. Treatment and Care Options

Medications and Therapies: There are medications available that can help manage symptoms, alongside therapies that support emotional and cognitive well-being.

Daily Care Strategies: Creating a supportive home environment and engaging in regular activities can enhance quality of life for individuals with dementia.

5. The Role of Diet in Managing Alzheimer's and Dementia

Brain-Healthy Foods: A diet rich in fruits, vegetables, whole grains, and healthy fats can support brain health.

Meal Planning: Encouraging healthy eating habits through practical meal planning can be beneficial for overall well-being.

6. Coping Strategies for Caregivers

Self-Care: Caregivers must prioritize their own well-being to provide the best care for their loved ones.

Support Networks: Connecting with support groups and resources can provide emotional and practical assistance.

7. Planning for the Future

End-of-Life Considerations: Discussing end-of-life wishes, funeral arrangements, and hospice care early on is crucial for ensuring that the individual's preferences are honored.

Ongoing Communication: Regular family discussions about care plans can enhance understanding and cooperation among family members.

Empowering Support and Resources

In addition to the insights shared in this guide, several resources can further support individuals, families, and caregivers affected by Alzheimer's and dementia.

Recommended Books

"The 36-Hour Day" by Nancy L. Mace and Peter V. Rabins: A comprehensive guide for families caring for those with Alzheimer's and dementia, offering practical advice and insights.

"Still Alice" by Lisa Genova: A novel that provides an intimate view of living with Alzheimer's, capturing the emotional and cognitive challenges faced by individuals and their families.

"Being Mortal" by Atul Gawande: This book explores the challenges of aging and end-of-life care, emphasizing the importance of quality of life.

"Creating Moments of Joy Along the Alzheimer's Journey" by Jolene Brackey: A guide focused on finding joy in daily life with loved ones affected by Alzheimer's.

Useful Websites

Alzheimer's Association: www.alz.org - A comprehensive resource offering information about Alzheimer's, caregiving tips, and support services.

Alzheimer's Society: www.alzheimers.org.uk - Provides information and support for individuals and families dealing with dementia.

National Institute on Aging: www.nia.nih.gov - Offers research-based information on aging, Alzheimer's, and related dementias.

Caregiver Action Network: www.caregiveraction.org - A resource for family caregivers, providing tips and support for managing caregiving challenges.

Support Organizations

Alzheimer's Foundation of America: Offers support groups, educational programs, and resources for individuals with dementia and their families.

Dementia Society of America: Provides resources, education, and support for families navigating dementia care.

AARP: Offers a wealth of resources for caregivers, including articles, forums, and webinars on various caregiving topics.

Final Thoughts

Navigating Alzheimer's and dementia can be challenging, but knowledge, planning, and support can make a significant difference. By understanding the conditions, recognizing early signs, and planning for the future, families can better prepare for the journey ahead.

Empowering oneself with the right resources and fostering open communication can help ensure that individuals affected by these conditions live fulfilling and dignified lives. Always keep in mind that you are not alone in this journey. Reach out, seek support, and stay informed. Together, we can build a community that embraces understanding, compassion, and resilience in the face of Alzheimer's and dementia.

Thank you for choosing to read this guide on Alzheimer's and dementia. Your feedback means the world to us, and we would love to hear your thoughts! Reviews play a crucial role in helping others find valuable resources and make informed choices. If this book has offered you insights, comfort, or support on your journey, please take a moment to share your honest review.

Your experience and opinions can truly make a difference, guiding others who may be facing similar challenges. Whether it's the personal stories that resonated with you, the practical advice that helped in caregiving, or even suggestions for improvement, we welcome all feedback.

Writing a review not only helps future readers but also motivates us to continue providing content that truly meets your needs. Thank you for being a part of this journey and for sharing your thoughts with us.

Printed in Dunstable, United Kingdom